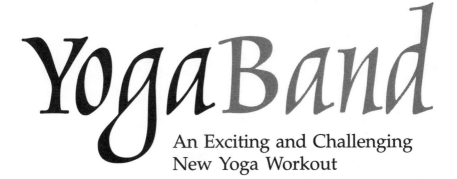

YogaBand

An Exciting and Challenging
New Yoga Workout

Lisa M. Wolfe

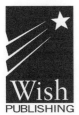

Wish Publishing
Terre Haute, Indiana
www.wishpublishing.com

LCCN: 2004104004

Editorial Assistance provided by Amanda Burkhardt and Heather Lowhorn
Cover designed by Phil Velikan
Photography provided by Lisa M. Wolfe

Printed in the United States of America
10 9 8 7 6 5 4 3 2 1

Published in the United States by
Wish Publishing
P.O. Box 10337
Terre Haute, IN 47801, USA
www.wishpublishing.com

Distributed in the United States by
Cardinal Publishers Group
7301 Georgetown Road, Suite 118
Indianapolis, Indiana 46268
www.cardinalpub.com

The YogaBand Workout Book is dedicated to my husband and two amazing children. Their daily support and encouragement of my path through fitness gives me the confidence needed to encourage others on the journey.

Table of Contents

Preface

Since yoga's increase to the number one trend for fitness participants, one would have to live in a cave to not have heard of yoga. Various books, videos, classes and magazine articles address this "new found" form of exercise.

Yoga consists of the physical postures, and also a life-style. The yoga philosophy can be found in many books, magazines, etc. What I am addressing here in this book, is a variation on the physical postures of yoga. I want you to bring your own philosophy to the workout. I encourage individuality in my children, friends, family and in my yoga class participants. I do not attempt to alter your life course, or your mind-set. My attempt here is to challenge your body in a unique way.

Your body will respond with increased strength, flexibility, and relaxation. You will also feel improved self-confidence knowing that your body can do anything you ask of it!

In your journey through health and wellness, you will make various stops along the way. Exercise and diet fads come and go. Choose the exercise program and eating habits that work the best for your body. Only you know what makes you feel good and healthy. Thank you for making this stop with me along your path. I hope this time with YogaBand is a successful one for you and that you will visit repeatedly!

In health,
Lisa

Introduction to the Popularity of Yoga

There are many reasons why the popularity of yoga has increased in recent years. Chief among these reasons are the needs and desires of an aging population seeking a more holistic approach to exercise. Fitness consumers are starting to feel the stress and bodily damage inflicted by years of high-impact workouts. Baby boomers are waking up each morning with new aches and pains in joints and lower backs. The younger population of fitness participants see the results of years of impact workouts on their older friends and family and seek an alternative. People everywhere are seeking a gentler way to exercise, while increasing the mind/body connection.

Yoga is a 5,000 year old Indian form of exercise. The goal of yoga is to unite the body and the mind. The word "Yoga" is a Sanskrit word meaning to yoke together, or unite. Yoga can become a way of life. Many yogis incorporate yogic principles into life choices; food, clothing, religion, etc. Yoga does not have to be taken to this extreme. In the West, yoga is most often associates with the physical yoga postures.

Over 100 different styles of yoga exist. Some of the most common styles: Raja yoga seeks to master and reject negative emotions, Mantra yoga uses chanting to achieve unity through sound, Iyengar yoga emphasizes perfecting poses with long holds, Bikram yoga is practiced in a VERY hot room, Ashtanga yoga or Power yoga, uses a series of poses in repetition to build heat, Hatha yoga is the style of yoga most common in the West. Hatha yoga uses physical postures in sequence with a flowing breath. YogaBand has it's foundations in Hatha yoga postures.

Various books and video tapes are available encouraging yoga exercise. Most cities and health clubs have yoga classes. Some even have the new hybrid classes such as "disco yoga" or yoga plus kickboxing. These hybrid classes are the result of the desire for change. Yoga runs the risk of giving way to the next new trend. To keep yoga fresh and challenging, we incorporate new elements into the basic yoga poses.

YogaBand adds a resistance element of a rubberized exercise band, increasing the strength training portion of a yoga session. When a muscle meets a new level of resistance, it responds to this increased force with added effort. This added effort, promotes muscle growth. The band adds variation and challenge to traditional yoga poses without taking away the yoga benefits.

The resistance bands are also used for increased range of motion in flexibility poses. We wrap the band around the feet, or hold in hands behind the back, to increase the flexibility in the legs and chest.

Another added benefit is the increased muscle usage, releases increased amounts of endorphins into the blood stream. Endorphins are the body's own natural pain killer hormones. These are the "feel good" hormones that give us that up lifted, happy feeling after exercise.

The addition of the band does not take away any of the benefits from traditional yoga. It does enhance the strength training, flexibility and relaxation phases of a yoga workout.

What is YogaBand?

The YogaBand Workout is a new journey through yoga. This workout uses exercise resistance bands to increase the strengthening, balancing, stretching and relaxing benefits of a yoga workout. The YogaBand workout combines familiar yoga poses such as Warrior I, Chair, and Lunge, with the new element of the resistance band to add challenge and intensity to your exercise program. The workout concludes with relaxation to calm and unite the body and mind.

The YogaBand workout is a way to motivate and challenge the body. YogaBand's benefits are similar to yoga. Some of the benefits seen are weight loss, cardiovascular conditioning, flexibility, increased energy level, increased self esteem, stress relief and an emphasis on strength gains. The band is added mainly to the strengthening poses, as opposed to the relaxation poses.

YogaBand uses rubberized resistance bands that are flat (4 to 6 inches wide), without handles and approximately 5-6 feet long. The bands can be purchased in rolls and cut to the correct length, or in sets of three at many sporting good stores. Exercise tubes provide resistance, but tend to roll out from under the foot. Latex-free bands are also available if you have latex allergies.

The bands come in various levels of resistance, differentiated by color. Choose the low to moderate resistance. This allows strength gains, while keeping the focus on the yoga breathing. Too much resistance and we begin to concentrate more on the body than on the breath. Have different levels available and practice with the band before a session to find the right comfort level for that day.

To properly care for the bands, store them in a small plastic bag, box, or hang in a dark area away from direct sunlight. Use caution if long fingernails or large rings will come into contact with the band. If the band gets punctured, it could snap. Talcum powder should be put into the bag periodically to help the band retain its elasticity.

Due to YogaBand's emphasis on strength gains, the workout should be performed every other day. The muscles of the body need a day of rest in between workouts to recover from the exercise. That way, the muscles will change and grow instead of breaking down and becoming susceptible to injuries. If the workout is practiced consistently, we will see results within four to six weeks. It takes that amount of time for the body to realize we are determined to stay with a workout and are serious about making changes.

The increased muscle tissue gained from the workout, increases metabolism. The muscles of the body burn calories 24 hours a day. So, even at rest, our muscle tissue is working for us! The more muscle tissue we have, the faster our metabolism.

Preparing for a Workout

The only equipment needed is your exercise band. A yoga mat is also helpful, as yoga mats are sticky, so feet and hands will not slip. Comfortable clothing should be worn to allow the body freedom of movement. Very tight clothing will restrict movement and very loose clothing may get in the way. Bare feet are preferred.

Find a quiet, uncluttered room without thick carpet to practice in. Thick carpet makes it difficult to balance. Choose a time when you will not be interrupted. Add your personal favorites to the workout such as soft music and candle light to ensure a successful yoga session. Practicing with music helps the mind to focus, allowing the body freedom of movement.

Yoga is best practiced on an empty stomach. Limit the amount of food intake for 1 1/2 hours before practicing yoga. You will want to have water available. A towel can also be nearby to wipe sweat, place under the knees for added comfort, or to cover the eyes in final relaxation.

Begin to clear your mind. When you step to the mat for your practice, BE there on the mat. Leave everything else off this mat and give yourself permission to let go of the real world for this time just for you. This might be difficult at first, but with practice, you will look forward to this quiet time.

Remember that there is no competition, no judgment and no expectations. Work with today's limitations of your body. Not every day will be the same and not each side of the body will be the same. Work with what you have now.

Embrace any feelings that surface while practicing yoga. It is not uncommon to laugh or to cry. Let yourself feel while you are in this quiet time. Physical sensations are common as well. Mild nausea, tingling sensations, headaches, dizziness or muscle cramps may occur. Over time these will subside. These are natural reactions to yoga. You choose how to respond. You may take a break, or try to work through the sensations.

The breathing is done solely through the nose. Focus the mind only on the breath. If the mind wanders, bring it back to the breath. Remember, to let everything else go. When the mind is focused on the breathing, it allows the body freedom to move. The mind is passive, while the body is active.

Reminders:
- Breathe only through the nose
- Practice on an empty stomach
- Focus on the breath
- Listen to the body and work within the limitations
- Be aware of feelings and allow yourself to feel

Special Considerations

Almost anyone can benefit from yoga. Since yoga challenges each body to its own limitations, even children can participate. The following special conditions should be given consideration before beginning the workout.

If you:
- are pregnant, please check with your doctor before beginning this or any exercise program. Do not place band around the stomach.
- have hypertension or high blood pressure, please check with your doctor. Avoid holding the breath, fully inverted poses, and holding the band too tightly. A lighter band resistance is recommended.
- have shoulder injuries or dislocations, a lighter resistance should be used.
- have lower back injuries, keep knees slightly bent during any forward bending
- have upper back injuries, do not drop the head back. Keep focus forward.
- have wrist pain, carpal tunnel syndrome, or arthritis in the hands, rest on the knuckles instead of the palms in kneeling poses, and keep wrists as straight as possible when working with the band.
- have a sensitivity to latex, wash hands immediately after using the bands, or purchase latex-free bands.
- are fatigued, listen to the body and adjust your practice for

the day.

- have a torn muscle or ligament, ease gently into the poses. Pull back from going all the way into a pose, until the injury is completely healed.
- have asthma, always carry your inhaler with you. If you have an attack during practice, stop.
- have diabetes, seek advice of your doctor, and have a snack on hand.

Breathing Technique

The MOST important element of any yoga workout is the breath. Breathe in and out through the nose. The added yoga band makes this breath work even more important. The descriptions will show the proper times to inhale and exhale. We breathe through the nose, but the breath comes from deeper underneath the chest and lungs. This area around the diaphragm should activate the inhale and exhale.

Traditional yoga believes that breath is the life force of the body. Think about it. Without breath there would be no life. We can learn to control the breath. Yoga uses slow and complete inhales and exhales. This controlled breath is remembered in the day to day life when we encounter a stressful situation. After a few moments of breathing, we feel calm and centered again.

Begin each session with a few minutes of quiet, controlled breath. Feel the oxygen traveling down through the neck, chest and stomach. Breathe into any tight areas of the body and as you exhale, release the tension. Focus the mind only on this breath. Remember, this is time for you.

Move into the yoga pose while inhaling. On an exhale, use a sinking breath to "sink" the body comfortably into the pose. You can hold the pose for a few breaths, or go right into the yogaband exercise.

The yogaband movements follow the complete breath, making the moves slow and controlled. On an inhale, expand the chest and the lungs completely. On an exhale, expel as much air out of the lungs as possible. As with all resistance training exercises, the exhale is on the exertion phase of the movement.

Safety Cautions when Using the Band

- Maintain the natural width of the band. This will allow for smoother movements, which will protect the joints.
- Hold the bands firm, but not too tightly; too tight a grip will impede blood flow in the arms and increase blood pressure.
- Use slow, controlled movements as opposed to jerking the bands.
- Adjust tension of the band at the beginning of each pose. Adequate tension in the muscles should be felt throughout the entire movement.
- Perform 8 to 10 repetitions of each exercise. You may begin by choosing 3-5 poses, until you are comfortable with a full hour of practice.
- Keep the spine straight and pull tight the abdominal muscles.
- Do not overextend any joints.
- Take a break when you need to.
- Flow through the workout slowly. Do not overstrain the body. If you are unable to complete a posture at first, take your time and sink as deep as you comfortably can. It is also beneficial to work the poses first without the band, adding the band in after the poses are mastered.

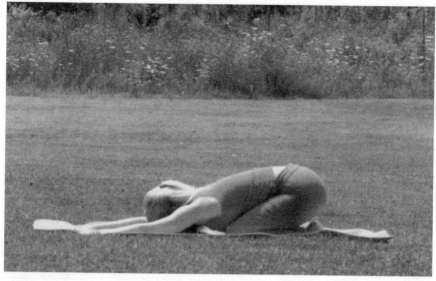

Photo 1

Extended Child's Pose

Beginning in Extended Child's Pose, we focus the breath. We breathe in through the nose and out through the nose. Here is where we begin to focus the mind on the breath. We let stray thoughts pass through the mind. Spend 4-5 minutes here, breathing and preparing the mind for the yoga session.

Getting into the pose:
- From hands and knees, sink the hips back onto the heels.
- Extend the arms out in front of the body, onto the mat.
- Palms pressing down with fingers spread like stars.
- Rest forehead onto the mat

Benefits:
- Stretches back and shoulders
- Relaxes mind and body

Modifications:
- If knee discomfort occurs, place padding under knees, or a rolled up towel in between the knees and calves.

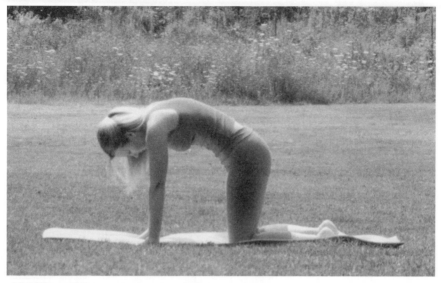

Photo 2

Cat/Cow Stretch

Cat/Cow is used to warm the spine, open the neck and continue focused breathing.

Getting into the pose:
- Come onto hands and knees.
- The wrists are directly under the shoulders.
- The knees are directly under the hips.
- Exhale and round the back, looking toward the feet. (Cat)
- Inhale and flex the back, looking straight ahead. (Cow)
- Continue alternating cat and cow, using the breath as the guide.

Benefits:
- Strengthens the neck, back, stomach, arms and shoulders.
- Stretches the back and stomach.

Modifications:

- If wrist discomfort occurs, place hands in fist, with knuckles on the floor.
- If knee discomfort occurs, place extra padding under knees.

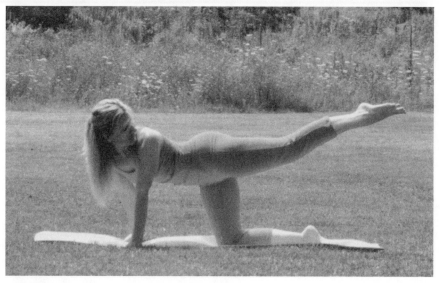

Photo 3

Spinal Balance With Backward Glance

Spinal Balance continues warming the body. It helps elongate the spine while strengthening the core muscles.

Getting into the pose:

- From all fours, inhale and lift a straight left leg, behind the body.
- Look back toward the left ankle.
- Keep the spine straight and the stomach pulled in tight.
- Exhale and lower the left leg.
- Inhale and lift the straight right leg.
- Exhale and lower.
- Using the breath, continue alternating sides of the body for 5-10 breath cycles.
- Concentrate on reaching away from the body through the toes.

- Work to lengthen the spine and maintain one long line from head to toe.

Benefits:

- Strengthens the back and core muscles of the body.
- Stretches the neck.

Modifications:

- Do not turn to look behind.
- Keep raised knee slightly bent.

Sun Salutations

Traditional yoga sun saluta-
tions are an excellent way to warm-
up the body. It is here that we gauge
how the body is feeling today. We
find any tight areas. Use a slow controlled breath to guide through the
poses. If you find that you want to
hold one pose for a few breaths, feel
free to do this. This is your time.
Listen to your body.

We begin in **Mountain Pose**
(Photo 4). Stand tall with feet hip
distance apart. Legs are straight.
Arms at sides, with palms facing
forward. The spine is straight with
the chin parallel to the floor. Begin
focused breathing.

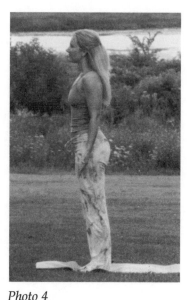

Photo 4

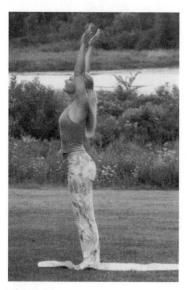

Photo 5

Inhale reaching **Arms Overhead** (Photo 5). Extend arms to the
sky, with outstretched fingers.
Look straight ahead, or slightly
bend backward looking up.

Exhale into **Airplane/Forward
Bend** (Photo 6 & 7). Bending forward from the waist, bring extended arms behind and to the side
of the body. Keep the spine
straight, then drop the hands onto
the mat for forward bend. Palms or
finger tips can be on the mat, or the
elbows can be on the knees.

Inhale stepping the right foot
to the back of the mat for a **Lunge**

18

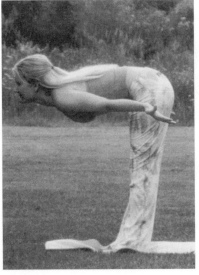

Photo 6

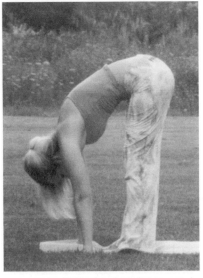

Photo 7

(Photo 8) remain on the toes of the right foot. Align the left knee over the left heel. Gently sink into the stretch, keeping the hands on the mat.

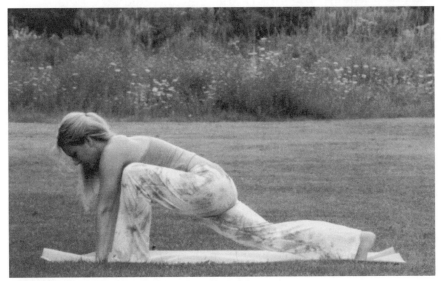

Photo 8

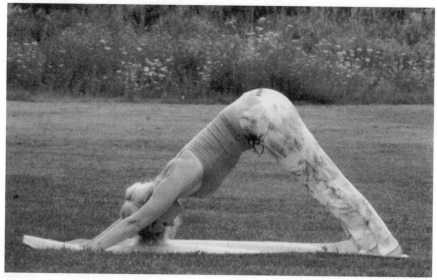

Photo 9

Exhale stepping the left foot to the back of the mat into **Downward Facing Dog** (Photo 9). The fingers are spread like stars. Extend the hips to the sky. Press the heels into the mat, the chest toward the tops of the legs and relax the neck.

Inhale, bringing the hips toward the mat and shoulders over the wrists into **Plank Pose** (Photo 10). The spine is straight and the stomach pulled in tight. Remain on the toes, sinking the hips, or bring the knees onto the mat.

Exhale into **Crocodile** (Photo 11). Bending the elbows, keeping the elbows next to the body bring the chest and head toward the mat. Keep the hips off of the mat.

Inhale, lower the hips and raise the chest and head into **Cobra** Keep the elbows slightly bent. Open the front of the body. For a more advanced version keep the hips off of the mat for **Upward Facing Dog** (Photo 12).

Exhale back into **Down Dog.** (Photo 9)

Inhale, step the right foot forward in between the hands into a **Lunge** (Photo 13). Remain on the toes of the left foot.

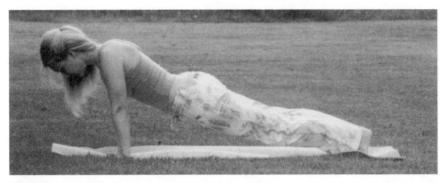

Photo 10

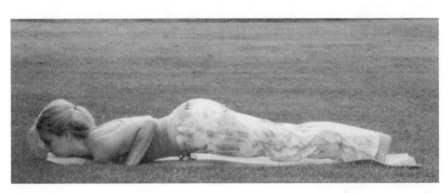

Photo 11

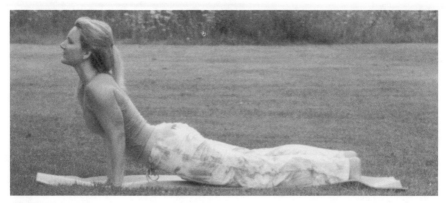

Photo 12

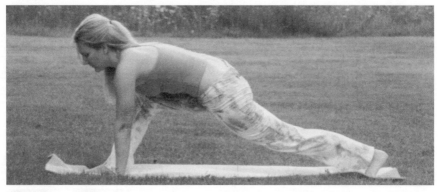

Photo 13

Align the right knee over the right heel. Gently sink into the stretch.

Exhale, step the left foot forward to the right for **Forward Bend** (Photo 7). Allow the top of the head to drop down.

Inhale, sink the hips, raise onto the fingertips and look forward for **Monkey Pose** (Photo 14).

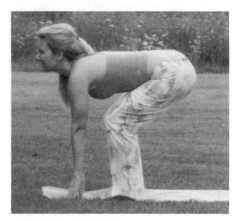

Photo 14

Exhale into **Chair** (Photo 15). Keep sinking the hips, bring the arms out in front of the body, or extend overhead. Keep the weight of the body on the heels. Keep the knees in line with the heels.

Inhale, reaching **Arms Overhead**.

Continue repeating 5-10 times depending on your needs for the day.

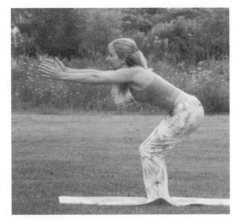

Photo 15

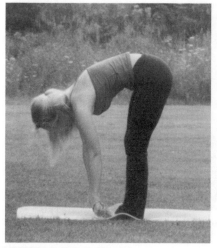

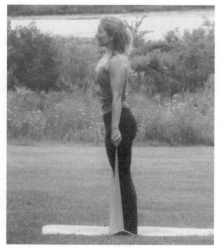

Photo 16   Photo 17

Forward Bend-Mountain-Forward Bend

Benefits:
- Strengthens and stretches the hamstrings and gluteals (back of the upper legs and butt).

- Strengthens and stretches the lower back.

Getting into the pose:
- Feet are hip distance apart.
- Position the middle of the band underneath both feet.
- Hold one end of the band in each hand.
- Take up the tension until the band is tight.
- Bend from the waist, allowing the top of the head to drop down into Forward Bend.
- Keep the legs straight and the stomach pulled in tight.

Breathing:
- Exhale, and stand straight up into Mountain pose.

- Arms are at sides.
- Inhale and lower back into Forward Bend.
- Repeat for desired number of repetitions.

Concentration:
- Focus on using the hamstrings and gluteals to pull body into standing position.
- Spine is straight and tall, chin parallel to the floor.
- Shoulders pulled down.

Modifications:
- Can keep knees slightly bent if any back pain occurs.
- Look forward throughout movement if neck pain occurs.

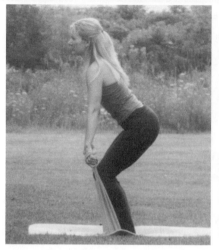

Photo 18

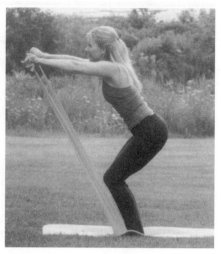

Photo 19

Chair With Front Deltoid Raise

Benefits:
- Strengthens legs, butt, back, feet, ankles and shoulders.

Getting into the pose:
- Stand with feet hip distance apart.
- Place middle of band underneath one or both (increased tension) feet.
- Hold one end of the band in each hand.
- Bend knees, sink hips toward the floor.

Breathing:
- Exhale, raising both straight arms, palms facing down, in front of the body up to eye level.
- Inhale, lowering arms next to the body.

Concentration:
- Focus on smooth movements.

- Keep knees over the heels.
- Weight of the body on the heels.
- Straight arms.
- Sink comfortably into the pose.

Modifications:

- Step the feet wider apart for stability and to avoid knee pain.
- Lift one arm at a time.

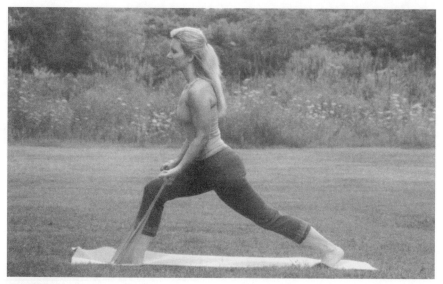

Photo 20

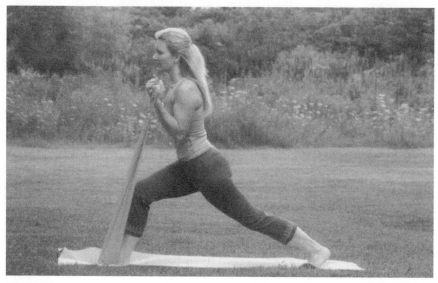

Photo 21

Standing Lunge With Bicep Curl

Benefits:
- Strengthens legs and biceps (front of upper arm).

Getting into the pose:
- Step the left foot to the back of the mat, remaining on toes.
- Bend right knee until approximately 90 degrees.
- Place middle of band underneath the right foot.
- Hold one end of band in each hand.
- Arms straight on both sides of right leg.

Breathing:
- Exhaling, bend arms at elbows and raise palms toward the shoulders.
- Inhaling, lower arms to the sides.

Concentration:
- Tighten the legs and biceps.
- Focus on a point straight ahead to maintain balance.
- Keep elbows tight against the body.
- Weight of the body on front heel.
- Keep knee over heel.
- Repeat on both legs.

Modifications:
- Curl one arm at a time.
- Place left heel onto mat for stability.
- Not sinking deeply into pose.

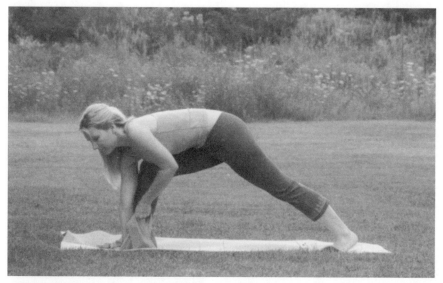

Photo 22

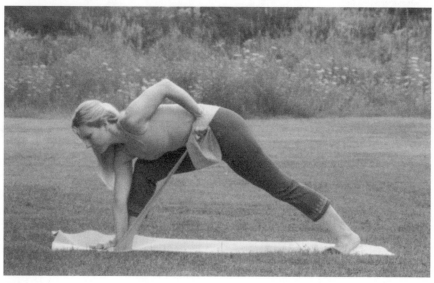

Photo 23

Extended Angle With Lat Pull In

Benefits:
- Slims waist.
- Stretches inner thighs and waist.
- Strengthens back, legs and glutes

Getting into the pose:
- Step left foot to back of mat, remaining on toes of left foot.
- Bend right knee to 90 degrees.
- Place right hand on mat near right foot.
- Place one end of band under right foot.
- Grasp end of band in left hand creating tension in band.

Breathing:
- Exhaling, pull left hand into left hip.
- Inhaling, release left hand down next to right ankle.

Concentration:
- Tighten the back.
- Focus on a point straight ahead.
- Keep elbow close to body.
- Elbow remains higher than hand.
- Keep elbow bent.
- Full range of motion.
- Repeat on both legs.

Modifications:
- Place left heel on the mat.
- Place right elbow on knee instead of hand on mat.

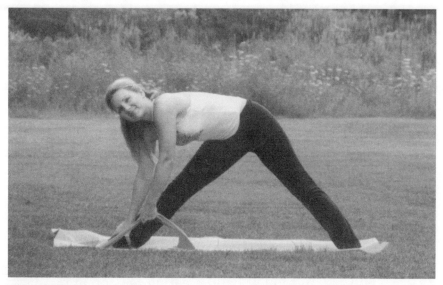

Photo 24

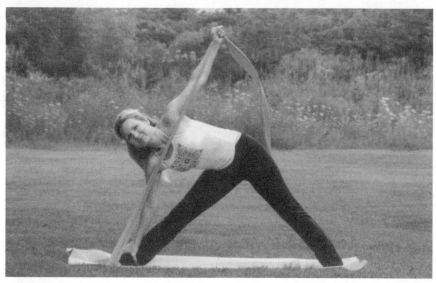

Photo 25

Triangle With Rear Deltoid

Benefits:
- Strengthens legs, torso and rear shoulder.
- Stretches waist and hamstrings.

Getting into the pose:
- Stand with arms parallel to the floor.
- Place feet wrist distance apart.
- Turn right foot out 90 degrees and left foot out 45 degrees.
- Align heel of right foot with arch of the left foot.
- Place one end of the band underneath the right foot.
- Straighten both legs.
- Bend from waist and place right hand on right ankle, or shin.
- Grasp the band in the left hand near the ankle, creating tension.
- Rest left arm alongside the right leg.
- Turn chest open.

Breathing:
- Exhale, extend straight left arm to sky opening the chest.
- Inhale, return arm alongside the right leg.

Concentration:
- Use the rear shoulder to move the arm.
- Look up, straight ahead or down.
- Press left shoulder backward.
- Keep legs and arms straight.
- Open front of body.
- Repeat on opposite leg.

Modifications:
- Placing the hand on a block or shin.
- Keeping the knees slightly bent.

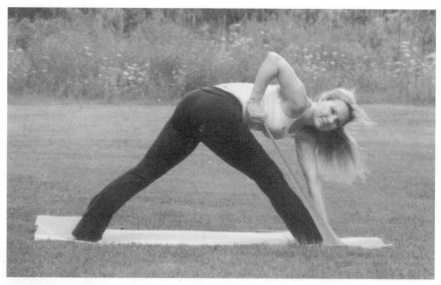

Photo 26

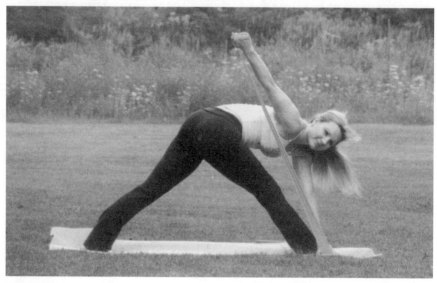

Photo 27

Reverse Triangle With Tricep Kickback

Benefits:
- Strengthens torso, legs and triceps (back of the upper arm).
- Stretches waist, back, hamstrings.

Getting into the pose:
- From triangle, rotate the upper body to place the left hand on the right ankle or on mat.
- Grasp the band in the right hand.
- Bend the right elbow, and raise the right hand to the right hip.

Breathing:
- Exhale, straighten the right arm behind the body.
- Inhale, and return the hand to the hip.

Concentration:
- Feel a contraction in the tricep with every extension.
- Look up, straight ahead or down.
- The elbow stays high above the body.
- Left shoulder presses forward.
- Right shoulder presses backward.
- Keep slight bend in elbow, never fully extend.
- Repeat on opposite leg.

Modifications:
- Bring hand to the mat on the inside of the right foot.
- Bring hand to the mat on the outside of the right foot for more advanced stretch.
- Bend knees slightly.

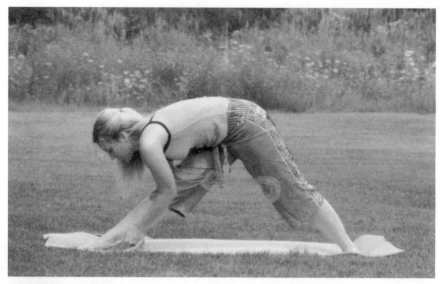

Photo 28

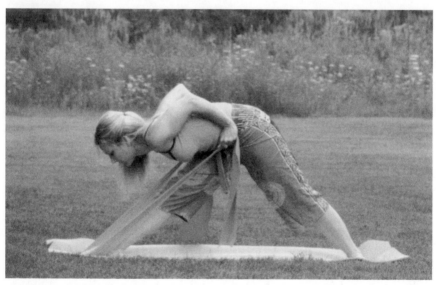

Photo 29

Pyramid Pose With Lat Pull-in

Benefits:
- Strengthens legs and back.
- Stretches hamstrings, lower back and hips.

Getting into the pose:
- Feet in same position as triangle.
- Middle of the band placed under the right (front) foot.
- Bend forward over the right leg.
- Drop the top of the head to face the ground.
- Hands placed on both sides of the right foot.
- Grasp one end of the band in each hand creating tension.

Breathing:
- Exhale, bending the arms, pulling both elbows close to the body, hands come to the hips.
- Inhale, and return arms next to the right leg.

Concentration:
- Hold stomach tight.
- Keep back straight.
- Squeeze shoulder blades together at top of movement.
- Keep elbows close to the body and higher than hands.
- Repeat on opposite leg.

Modifications:
- Keep knees slightly bent.
- Place hands on shins instead of floor.
- Pull one arm in at a time.

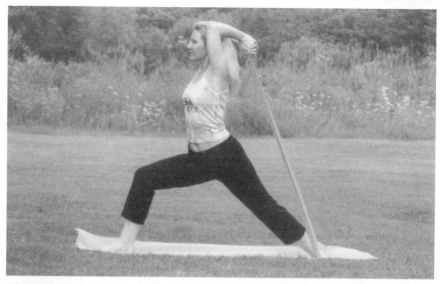

Photo 30

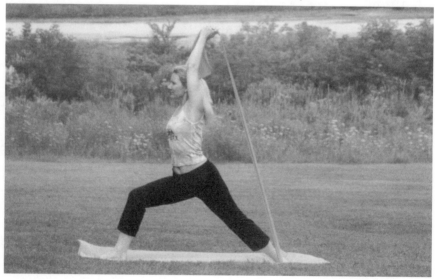

Photo 31

Warrior I With Overhead Tricep Extension

Benefits:
- Strengthens quads, glutes and triceps.
- Stretches back and hips.

Getting into the pose:
- Same feet position as triangle.
- Place one end of the band underneath the ball of left (back) foot.
- Take other end of the band into both hands.
- Bend right knee to a comfortable angle, not exceeding 90 degrees.
- Straighten left leg.
- Hold hands behind head with elbows bent, keeping elbows close to ears.

Breathing:
- Exhale, extend arms to the sky.
- Inhale, return arms to bent behind head.

Concentration:
- Contract triceps.
- Look forward or slightly up.
- Weight of front foot on the heel.
- Elbows remain close to head.
- Shoulders pull down away from ears.
- Sink comfortably into the pose.
- Pull stomach in tight and keep your back straight.
- Repeat on opposite leg.

Modifications:
- Slightly bend back knee.
- Hold onto band with one hand at a time for more advanced.

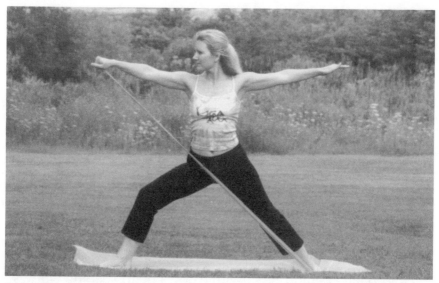

Photo 32

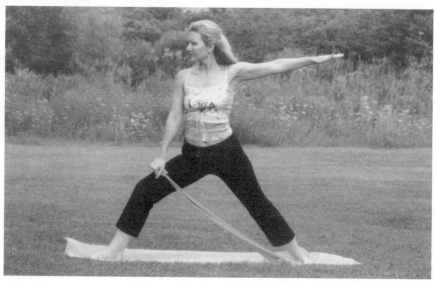

Photo 33

Warrior II With Lateral Shoulder Raise

Benefits:
- Strengthens quads, glutes, shoulders.
- Stretches chest and inner thigh.

Getting into the pose:
- Same feet as triangle.
- Place one end of band underneath the ball of the left (back) foot.
- Hold other end of band in right hand.
- Extend arms out at shoulder height.

Breathing:
- Inhale, lowering straight right arm in front of the body.
- Exhale, lifting the right arm to shoulder height.

Concentration:
- Look out over the right hand.
- Do not lift arm any higher than shoulder level.
- Sink comfortably into the pose.
- Weight of body on front heel.
- Repeat on opposite leg.

Modifications:
- Slightly bend back knee.
- Lower back arm.

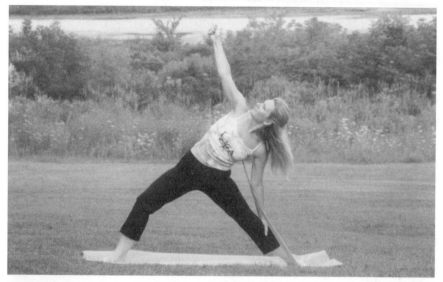

Photo 34

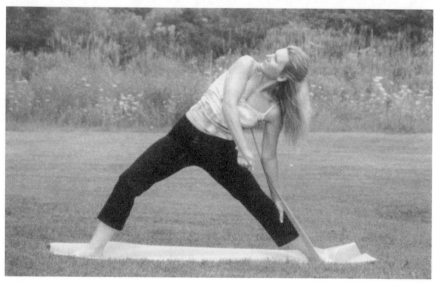

Photo 35

Reverse Warrior With Chest Fly

Benefits:
- Strengthens quads, glutes, pecs (chest).
- Stretches inner thighs, waist and back.

Getting into the pose:
- Same feet as triangle.
- Place one end of band underneath the left (back) foot.
- Take hold of other end of band in right hand, band traveling across back.
- Keep arms straight as the left hand travels down the left leg to a comfortable position.
- The right arm is straight up toward the sky holding band tight.

Breathing:
- Exhaling, lower right straight arm across front of body, closing chest.
- Inhaling, raise right arm to beginning position.

Concentration:
- Contract the chest as the arms close together.
- Concentrate on moving the elbow completely through the movement.
- Look up or straight ahead.
- Keep front knee over heel.
- Lengthen through the rib cage.
- Square hips to the side.
- Rest back hand above or below, not directly on the knee.
- Repeat on opposite leg.

Modifications:
- Keep back leg slightly bent.
- Do not sink deeply into the pose.

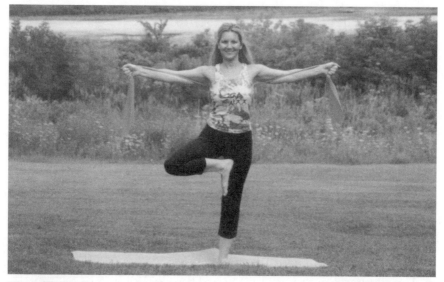

Photo 36

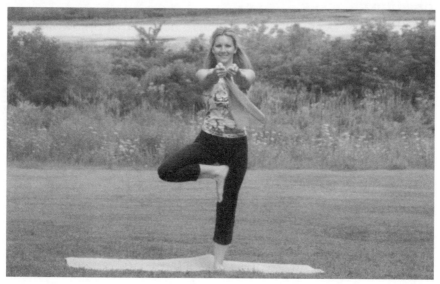

Photo 37

Tree Pose With Chest Fly

Benefits:
- Strengthens glutes, quads, chest and arms.
- Stretches inner thighs and back.

Getting into pose:
- Stand in center of mat.
- Feet hip distance apart.
- Wrap band behind back, holding one end of band in each hand, with band resting underneath the arms.
- Shift weight onto right leg.
- Place arch of left foot on right ankle, calf or inner thigh, avoiding the knee.
- Extend arms out to sides at shoulder height.

Breathing:
- Exhale, close arms together in front of body.
- Inhale, open arms out to sides.

Concentration:
- Find a stable focal point to concentrate on.
- Bring the elbows together in the middle of the movement, for chest contraction.
- Use enough tension to feel contraction.
- Keep elbows slightly bent.
- Maintain arms at shoulder height.
- Repeat on opposite leg.

Modifications:
- One arm at a time
- Keep left toes on floor for more balance.

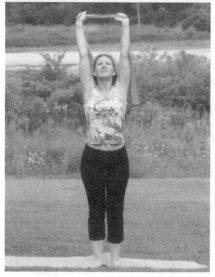

Photo 38

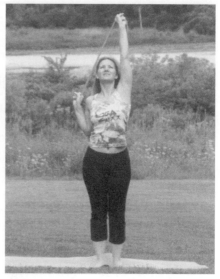

Photo 39

Side Lateral Stretch With Lat Pull-down

Benefits:
- Strengthens waist and lats (back).
- Stretches back and sides.

Getting into the pose:
- Stand with feet hip distance apart.
- Legs and back are straight.
- Hold toward the middle of the band with both hands.
- Tighten band tension.
- Extend arms straight overhead.

Breathing:
- Exhale, bend the right elbow, pulling the right arm down to the side.
- Inhale, return arm overhead.

- Exhale, bend the left elbow, pulling the left arm down to the side.
- Inhale, return arm overhead.

Concentration:
- Pull elbows down into the sides.
- Stand tall with stomach pulled in and back straight.
- Slight bend in the knees, do not lock the joints.
- Contract the back when pulling the elbow down.

Modifications:
- Slightly bend knees.
- Instead of alternating, execute total number of repetitions on one side then the other.

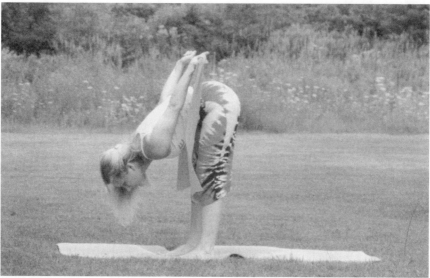

Photo 40

Standing Chest Expansion (Stretch)

Benefits:
- Stretches chest, lower back and hamstrings.

Getting into the pose:
- Stand with feet hip distance apart.
- Hold the middle of the band with both hands near the small of the back.

Breathing:
- Exhaling, fold out forward into forward bend.
- Extend straight arms out behind body, expanding the chest.
- Compete inhale and exhale through the nose.

Concentration:
- Top of the head drops down.

- Look behind, or eyes closed.
- Use as much tension as possible, to open the front of the body.
- Hold for 5 breaths.

Modifications:
- Keep knees slightly bent if back pain occurs.

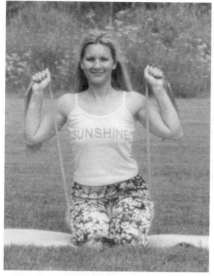

Photo 41

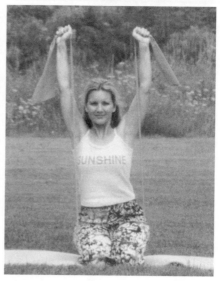

Photo 42

Hero Pose With Shoulder Press

Benefits:
- Strengthens shoulders and back.
- Stretches legs.

Getting into the pose:
- Sit with knees bent and feet underneath hips.
- Place middle of band under hips between hips and legs.
- Hold one end of band in each hand.
- Back is straight.
- Bring arms up, bent at elbows with hands next to shoulders, palms facing away.

Breathing:
- Exhale and extend arms toward the sky, keeping palms facing away from body.

- Inhale and lower arms bringing the hands in line with shoulders.

Concentration:
- Look forward.
- Complete range of motion.
- Bring hands back down to shoulder level.

Modifications:
- If knee pain, place a rolled up towel behind knees or place band between knees and mat and lift hips off of knees.
- Raise one arm at a time.

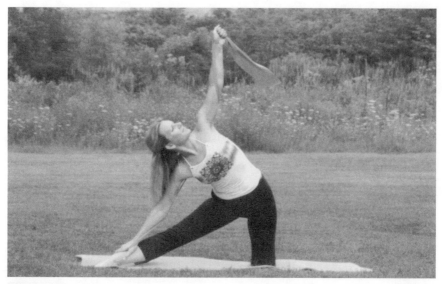

Photo 43

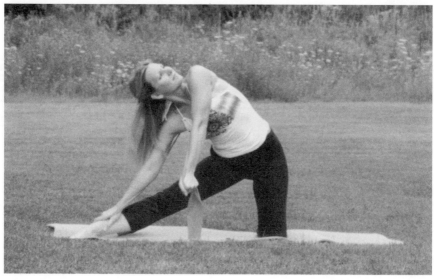

Photo 44

Gate With Chest Fly

Benefits:
- Strengthens outer and inner thighs and chest.
- Stretches torso and hips.

Getting into the pose:
- Begin on knees.
- Middle of band is behind back.
- Take hold of one end of band in each hand.
- Extend right leg out to the side.
- Slide right hand down right leg.
- Extend left straight arm up toward the sky.

Breathing:
- Exhaling, lower left straight arm toward the right, closing the chest.
- Inhaling, raise left arms toward the sky.

Concentration:
- Look straight ahead, up or down.
- Focus on contracting the chest.
- Squeeze the elbow toward the opposite arm.
- Elbows slightly bent.
- Repeat on opposite leg.

Modifications:
- Place a towel under the knees.
- Do not sink deeply into the pose.

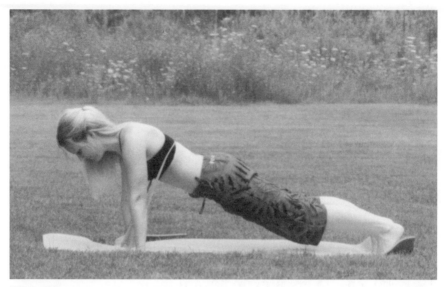

Photo 45

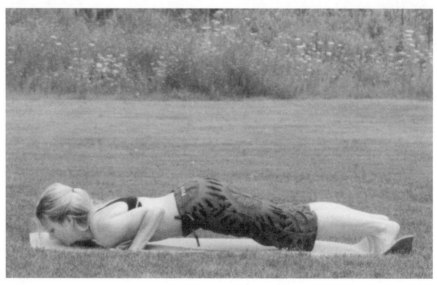

Photo 46

Plank-Crocodile-Plank

Benefits:
- Strengthens chest, arms, gluteals and core.

Getting into the pose:
- Wrap middle of band around back.
- Hold one end of band in each hand.
- Place hands on mat directly underneath shoulders.
- Begin on hands and knees.
- Straighten legs and raise onto toes.
- Sink the hips slightly toward the ground.

Breathing:
- Inhale, and lower the chest, head and hips toward the ground, keeping the elbows in close to the body.
- Exhale, straightening the arms back to the start.

Concentration:
- Keep the hips down and elbows close to the body.
- Hold stomach tight and back straight.
- Sink hips toward the mat, without sagging the back.
- Elbows stay close to the body.
- Work with the pace of the breath.

Modifications:
- Lowering the knees to the ground.
- On fists instead of palms.

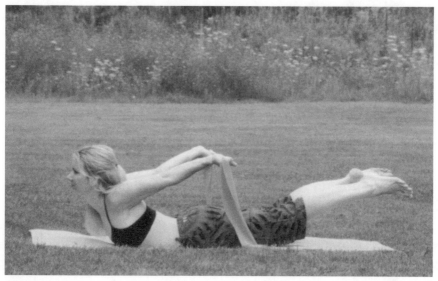

Photo 47

Locust Pose With Chest Expansion (Stretch)

Benefits:
- Strengthens back of body.
- Stretches chest and front of legs.

Getting into the pose:
- Lie face down.
- Grasp middle of band in both hands at small of back.

Breathing:
- Inhaling, lift head, chest, legs and arms toward the sky.
- Hold for 5 complete breaths.

Concentration:
- Look forward.
- Open front of body.

- Lift hands to a comfortable height.
- Bring shoulder blades together.
- Squeeze buttocks.
- Reach away from the center of body with arms and legs.

Modifications:
- Not lifting arms, legs and chest as high.

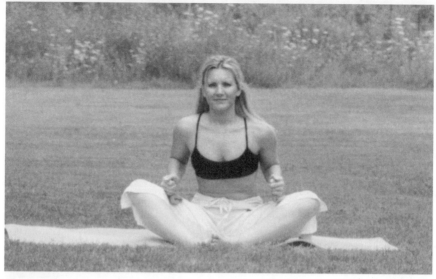

Photo 48

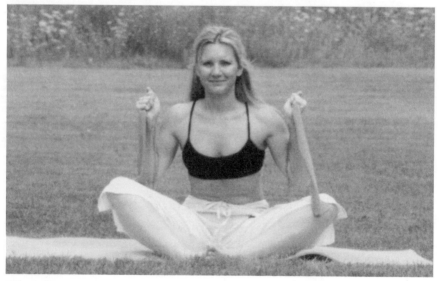

Photo 49

Butterfly With Hammer Curls

Benefits:
- Strengthens biceps.
- Stretches hips, groin and lower back.

Getting into pose:
- Sit in center of mat with back straight.
- Sit on the middle of the band.
- Hold one end of the band in each hand, creating tension.
- Bring soles of feet together in front of body.
- Press knees toward the floor.
- Keep arms straight at sides of body with palms facing each other.

Breathing:
- Exhale, bend elbows lifting fists toward the shoulders.
- Inhale, lower arms back to sides.

Concentration:
- Focus straight ahead.
- Full range of motion.
- Chin parallel to the floor.
- Keep palms facing each other.

Modifications:
- Sit on a small blanket or rolled up towel.
- Move feet further away from body.

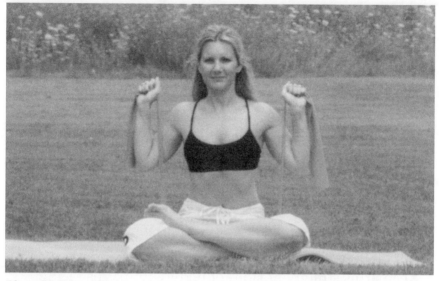

Photo 50

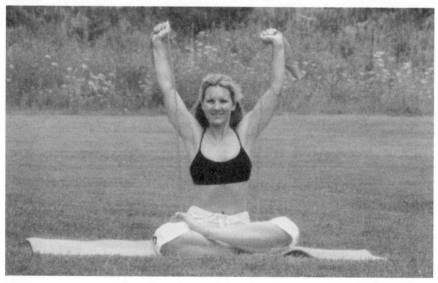

Photo 51

Lotus Pose With Shoulder Press

Benefits:
- Stretches legs.
- Strengthens shoulders and back.

Getting into the pose:
- Sit with legs crossed.
- Sit on middle of band.
- Gently lift right foot and place it on left thigh.
- Gently lift left foot and place it on right thigh.
- Take hold of one end of band in each hand.
- Bring palms to shoulder level with elbows down.

Breathing:
- Exhaling, extend arms straight up toward the sky.
- Inhaling, release palms down to shoulders, keeping elbows low.

Concentration:
- Sit up tall.
- Press through full shoulder range of motion.
- Chin parallel to floor.
- Elbows remain lower than hands.

Modifications:
- A half lotus seated pose instead. One leg up on opposite thigh.
- Sitting cross legged on floor.
- Placing a rolled up towel or blanket underneath body.
- Raising one arm at a time.

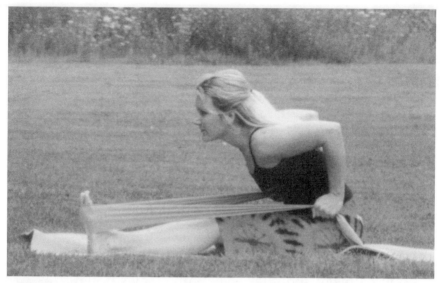

Photo 52

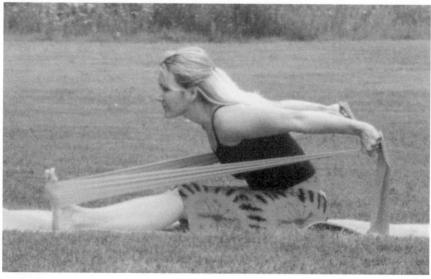

Photo 53

Seated Forward Fold With Tricep Kickback

Benefits:
- Stretches hamstrings, lower back and calves.
- Strengthens triceps.

Getting into the pose:
- Sit with legs straight in front of body.
- Place both feet on middle of band.
- Take hold of one end of band in each hand.
- Fold forward from the hips, pressing the chest into the legs.
- Bend elbows, bringing hands to hips and elbows behind body.

Breathing:
- Exhaling, extend arms straight behind body.
- Inhaling, return to bent elbows.

Concentration:
- Allow top of head to drop down.
- Focus on breath.
- Slow and controlled extension of arms.
- Elbows remain higher than hands.
- Feel contraction in triceps when extending arms.

Modifications:
- Bend the knees if any pain in back.
- Can sit on a rolled up towel or blanket.
- Look forward instead of down.
- Move one arm at a time through exercise.

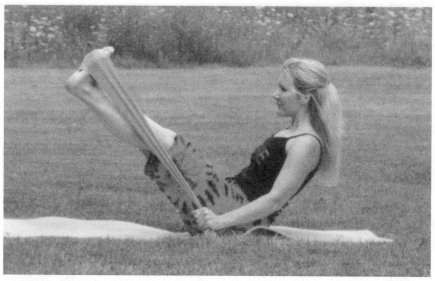

Photo 54

Boat Pose

Benefits:
- Strengthens torso, quads and hip flexors.
- Stretches Hamstrings.

Getting into the pose:
- Sitting with legs straight out in front of body.
- Place feet on middle of band.
- Hold ends of band in each hand.

Breathing:
- Exhale, lifting feet off of the mat.
- Complete inhale and exhale while balancing on sit bones.

Concentration:
- Focus on a stable point.

- Hold steady.
- Find the balancing point on the sit bones.
- Use the band's tension to help keep legs elevated.
- Hold stomach in tight.

Modifications:

- Bend the knees and wrap band around knees.
- Lift legs higher toward the sky.

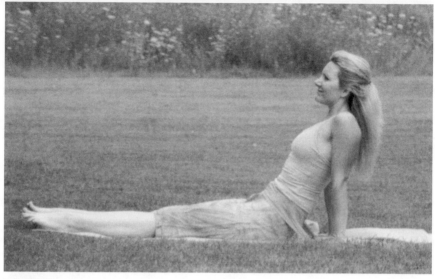

Photo 55

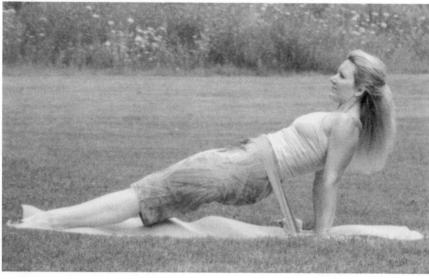

Photo 56

Incline Plank

Benefits:
- Strengthens arms, glutes, hamstrings, torso.
- Stretches chest, shoulders, hip flexors and abdominals.

Getting into the pose:
- Sitting with straight legs in front of body.
- Place middle of band around waist.
- Hold ends of band in hands.
- Hands placed on the mat with fingers pointing toward the feet.
- Point the toes.

Breathing:
- Exhaling, lift hips toward the ceiling.
- Can hold for 5 breaths, or inhaling release hips toward the mat.
- Repeat for repetitions.

Concentration:
- Open front of body.
- Keep hips elevated.
- Look forward or slightly up.
- Palms are flat with fingers pointing toward the feet.
- Feet are pointed.
- Straighten arms at top of movement.
- Squeeze shoulder blades together.
- Hold stomach tight.
- Keep spine straight.

Modifications:
- Bend knees.
- Come onto fists if pain in wrists occurs.

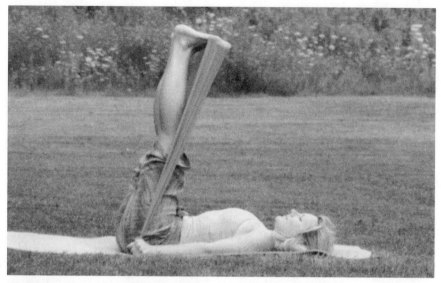

Photo 57

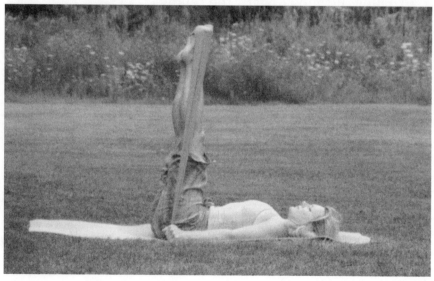

Photo 58

Upward Raised Legs With Calf Press

Benefits:
- Stretches and strengthens legs.
- Stretches lower back.

Getting into the pose:
- Lying on back, extend both straight legs toward the sky.
- Place middle of the band around bottoms of feet.
- Hold one end of the band in each hand.
- Create tension by pulling the hands closer to the body.
- Rest hands on the mat.

Breathing:
- Exhale and extend the toes.
- Inhale, and flex the foot.
- Repeat for repetitions.

Concentration:
- Press lower back into the mat.
- Press toes into band to prevent slipping.
- Neck stays still.
- Create comfortable tension for resistance in calves.

Modifications:
- Keep knees slightly bent.

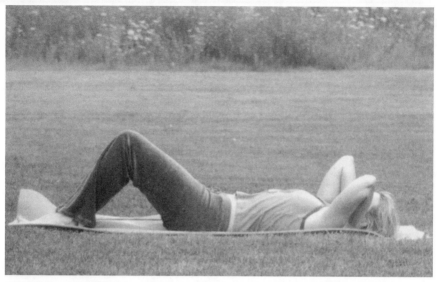

Photo 59

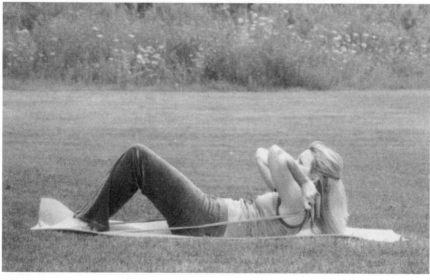

Photo 60

Trunk Flexion

Benefits:
- Strengthens abdominals, obliques (sides) and hip flexors.

Getting into the pose:
- Lying on back with knees bent.
- Place middle of band underneath feet.
- Hold one end of the band in each hand.
- Loop band under the body, holding onto the ends with hands next to the shoulders.
- Keep the spine straight and the stomach pulled in.
- Tilt the hips so that the lower back is resting on the floor.

Breathing:
- Exhale, lifting the chest toward the sky, shoulder blades coming up off of the mat.
- Inhale, lowering the shoulder blades back onto the mat.

Concentration:
- Press toes into band for stability.
- Stomach pulled in tight.
- Back pressed into mat.
- Look toward the sky and keep neck still.

Modifications:
- Widen the feet if any discomfort in the knees.

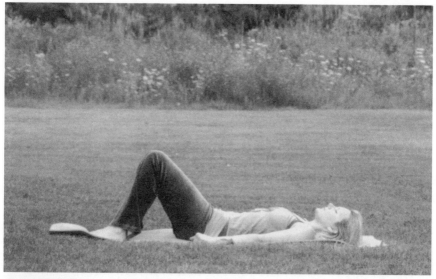

Photo 61

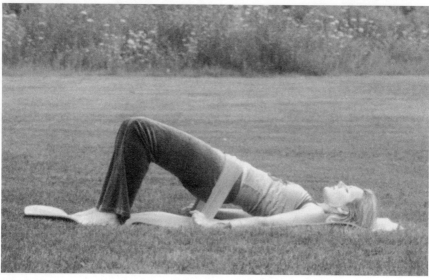

Photo 62

Bridge

Benefits:
- Strengthens gluteals, hamstrings and calves.
- Stretches abdominals, lower back and chest.

Getting into the pose:
- Lie on back with knees bent and feet on ground.
- Place middle of band across hips.
- Hold one end of band in each hand creating tension.
- Place hands on mat next to hips.
- Keep the head and neck very still.

Breathing:
- Exhale and lift hips toward the sky.
- Inhale and lower hips to ground.

Concentration:
- Press hips as high as possible.
- Hold neck still.
- Feet parallel.
- Use breath to open the body.

Modifications:
- Widen feet distance if any knee pain.
- Can be held static at top of movement.

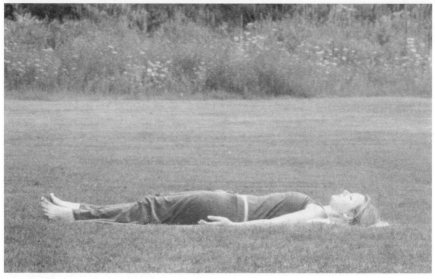

Photo 63

Final Relaxation

The goal of yoga is to unite the body and the mind. At the end of every session, we need quiet time for this to occur. Lie on your back, legs straight on ground, arms at sides with palms facing up and close your eyes. Begin focusing the mind on the breath. If a stray thought comes into the mind, let it pass as if floating off on a cloud during a windy day.

The eyes are closed gently. The muscles of the face are relaxed with the jaw slightly open. Feel the relaxation travel down the neck and over both shoulders that are resting comfortably on the ground. The tops of the arms are relaxed, the elbows slightly bent, the backs of the hands resting on the ground and the fingers are slightly curled in.

The chest is expanding with every breath, as you take the oxygen deep down into the stomach. The lower back is loose and the hips are open. Feel that relaxation travel down the tops of the legs, over the front and back of the knees, through the calves, ankles, feet and surrounding the toes.

Let yourself be surrounded with peace and calm. Take these moments just for you. Listening to your breath. You've worked hard today and you deserve this!

Remember how important you are and how important your needs are. Take care of yourself and enjoy your journey.

Sample Practice Format (One Hour)

Suggested flow

(Warm-up)

    Relaxation pose- focused breathing

    Bridge pose- band on waist

    Knees to chest- roll up into seated position

    Boat pose- band on feet

    Incline plank- band on waist

    Cat/Cow

    Downward Facing Dog

(Banded workout)

    Right leg lunge with bicep curl

    Triangle with rear delt

    Pyramid with lat pull-in

    Reverse Triangle with tricep kickback

    Forward Bend-Mountain-Forward Bend

    Chair with side lateral raise

    Left leg lunge with hammer bicep curl

    Triangle with rear delt

    Pyramid with lat pull-in

    Reverse Triangle with tricep kickback

    Forward bend-grasp middle of band with both hands

Inhale arms overhead to Side lateral stretch with lat pull-down

Tree with chest fly- left and right leg

Forward bend with chest expansion

Downward facing Dog

Plank

Crocodile

Cobra

Plank-Crocodile-Plank with band around back

Locust holding band at small of back to expand chest

Down Dog

Right leg lunge

Side straddle to place band underneath back foot (left)

Warrior I with tricep overhead extension

Warrior II with side lateral shoulder raise

Reverse Warrior with rear delt (drop band)

Hands down to front of mat, Step back to Down Dog

Sit into Lotus pose band under body for shoulder press

Onto knees right leg gate pose with chest fly

Left leg gate pose with chest fly

Place band under right foot, step left forward to lunge

Warrior I with tricep overhead extension

Warrior II with side lateral shoulder raise

Reverse Warrior with rear delt (drop band)

Hands to front of mat, step forward into Forward Bend

Cross legs, sink hips onto mat for butterfly pose, band under body, reverse bicep

Straighten legs, band around feet, roll down into trunk flexion

Upward raised legs with calf press

(Cool- Down)

Knees to chest

Circle knees

Final relaxation- guided meditation, positive reinforcement

Energizing routine

Sun salutation warm-up

Hold in Crocodile

Crocodile-Plank-Crocodile

Down Dog to Forward bend

Forward bend-mountain-forward bend

Chair with side shoulder raise

Arms overhead with pull down

Tree with chest fly

Warrior I with Tricep extension

Warrior II with Shoulder raise

Lunge with bicep curl

Repeat from Forward bend-Mountain-Forward bend on opposite leg

Finish with a few minutes of quiet breath in Mountain Pose.

More Information...

To Purchase Clothes Featured in Photos:
Yoga Chixx www.yogachixx.com, yogachix11@hotmail.com
Marika www.marika.com

For further information:
YogaFit Training Systems 310-376-1036, 888-786-3111
www.yogafit.com
Yoga Alliance 877-964-2255
www.yogaalliance.org
www.yogazone.com 800-264-9642
Yoga Journal 510-841-9200
www.yogajournal.com
www.yogasite.com

To Purchase Yoga Products:
www.yogaaccessories.com 800-990-9642
www.yogapro.com 800-488-8414
www.fitnesswholesale.com 800-396-7337
www.gaiam.com 800-254-8464
www.spriproducts.com 800-222-7774
www.huggermugger.com 800-473-4888

Author Biography

Lisa M. Wolfe has an Associates Degree in Exercise Science, is an ACE (American Council on Exercise) certified personal trainer and group fitness instructor, is a YogaFit certified instructor, has fourteen years of experience in the fitness industry including owning her own gym and is a freelance fitness writer for various magazine publications.

Visit *www.yogaband.com*, or e-mail *yogaband@hotmail.com* to reach Lisa M. Wolfe or purchase the YogaBand™ video series.

Also Available from Wish Publishing

Complete Conditioning for the Female Athlete
O'Connor, Fasting, Dahm and Wells
"What distinguishes this volume from so many lesser works is its research...This is a wonderful reference for any coach..." –Oxygen Magazine
WISH PUBLISHING • $18.95 • 320 pages • 7 x 10 photos • ISBN 1-930546-47-5 • trade paper • Ctn. Qty: 18

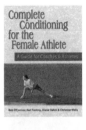

The Female Athlete: Train for Success
Bradley, Brzycki, Carlson, Harrison, Picone & Wakeham
A comprehensive and user-friendly guide to increasing female athlete performance.
WISH PUBLISHING • $16.95 • 256 pages • 7 x 10 ISBN: 1-930546-67-X • trade paper • photos • Ctn. Qty: 34

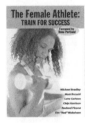

Total Fitness for Women
Joe Luxbacher, Leslie Bonci and Kim King
Clearly demonstrates how each of us possess the power to control and shape our own bodies.
WISH PUBLISHING • $14.95 • 160 pages • 5½ x 8½ illus. • ISBN: 1-930546-55-6 • trade paper • Ctn. Qty: 80

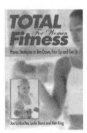

Female Fitness on Foot
O'Connor, Enoksen, Wells and Onsgard
Get the most out of your fitness regime. This book covers running, jogging, walking and orienteering. Reviewed in *Oxygen, Library Journal* and *Choice*.
WISH PUBLISHING • $16.95 • 256 pages • 7 x 10 ISBN: 1-930546-52-1 • trade paper • photos • Ctn. Qty: 24

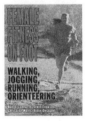

Wish Publishing's titles are available from quality bookstores nationwide or by calling (812) 299-5700

Also Available from Wish Publishing

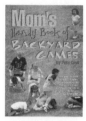

Mom's Handy Book of Backyard Games
Pete Cava
WISH PUBLISHING • $9.95 • 128 pages • 5½ x 8½
ISBN: 1-930546-43-2 • trade paper • photos • Ctn. Qty: 108

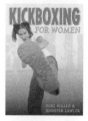

Kickboxing for Women
Jennifer Lawler and Debz Buller
Covers all the essentials of learning kickboxing, with tips especially for women.
WISH PUBLISHING • $16.95 • 256 pps • 7 x 10 • photos
ISBN 1-930546-53-X • trade paper • Ctn Qty: 40

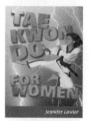

Tae Kwon Do For Women
Jennifer Lawler
"Finally! What took so long? Jennifer Lawler has written a book that was long overdue..." — TAEKWONDO magazine
WISH PUBLISHING • $16.95 • 256 pages • 7 x 10 • photos
ISBN: 1-930546-44-0 • trade paper • Ctn Qty: 24

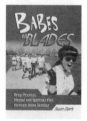

Babes on Blades
Suzan Davis
A lively in-line skating how-to for baby booming women and a personal journal of empowerment in the "Babe" way.
WISH PUBLISHING • $16.95 • 256 pages • 5½ x 8½
ISBN: 1-930546-54-8 • trade paper • photos • Ctn. Qty: 68

Wish Publishing's titles are available from quality bookstores nationwide or by calling (812) 299-5700